AGING WITH ELEGANCE

Inspiring Women to Embrace Their Years

A.C. Stallings RN

independent

Cover design by: Art Painter
Library of Congress Control Number: 2018675309
Printed in the United States of America

INTRODUCTION

Ladies, our journey through life is filled with highs and lows, victories and obstacles. As we age, it's crucial to approach the process gracefully and with acceptance. In the captivating subchapter "Embracing the Journey of Aging" from the inspiring book "Aging with Elegance: Inspiring Women to Embrace Their Years," we explore the power of embracing the changes that come with age and how it can empower us to live life to the fullest.

Aging is a natural part of life, and instead of fearing it, we should embrace it. By accepting the internal and external changes, we open ourselves up to new possibilities and experiences. This subchapter focuses on the importance of letting go of societal expectations and embracing the unique beauty and wisdom that comes with age.

Taking care of our physical and mental well-being is a key aspect of aging gracefully. This subchapter provides practical advice on maintaining a healthy lifestyle, including exercise, nutrition, and self-care routines. It also emphasizes the significance of nurturing our mental health through mindfulness practices and finding purpose and fulfillment in our daily lives.

Table of Contents
Chapter 1: The Beauty of Aging

Chapter 2: Cultivating Inner Strength

Chapter 3: Nurturing Relationships and Connections

Chapter 4: Embracing Beauty at Any Age

Aging with Elegance:

Inspiring Women to Embrace Their Years

A.C. Stallings RN

CHAPTER 1: THE BEAUTY OF AGING

Embracing the Journey of Aging

As women, our journey through life is filled with ups and downs, triumphs, and challenges. And as we grow older, it is important to approach the process of aging with grace and acceptance. In the subchapter titled "Embracing the Journey of Aging" from the book "Aging with Elegance: Inspiring Women to Embrace Their Years," we explore the significance of embracing the changes that come with age and how it can empower us to live our lives to the fullest.

Aging is a natural part of life, and instead of dreading it, we should strive to embrace it. By accepting the changes that occur both internally and externally, we open ourselves up to new possibilities and experiences. This subchapter delves into the importance of letting go of societal expectations and embracing the unique beauty and wisdom that comes with age.

One of the key aspects of aging gracefully is taking care of our physical and mental well-being. This subchapter offers practical advice on maintaining a healthy lifestyle, including exercise, proper nutrition, and self-care routines. It also emphasizes the significance of nurturing our mental health through mindfulness practices and finding purpose and fulfillment in our daily lives.

Furthermore, this subchapter explores the importance of cultivating a positive mindset and self-compassion. It highlights the power of reframing negative thoughts and focusing on self-acceptance and self-love. By embracing who we are at every stage of life, we can radiate confidence and inspire others to follow suit.

The journey of aging is not without its challenges, and this subchapter acknowledges that. It guides navigating common issues such as changes in relationships, transitioning into retirement, and finding new passions and hobbies. By sharing inspiring stories and practical advice from women who have embraced their years, readers are encouraged to face these challenges with resilience and optimism.

Ultimately, "Embracing the Journey of Aging" reminds women that age is just a number, and it should never define our worth or limit our dreams. By embracing the changes that come with aging and letting go of societal pressures, we can truly live our lives with elegance, grace,

and fulfillment. This subchapter serves as a guide and a source of inspiration for women to embrace their years and age with confidence and joy.

ACCEPTING THE PASSAGE OF TIME

In the journey of life, time is an unstoppable force that spares no one. As women, we often find ourselves caught in a whirlwind of responsibilities and expectations. We strive to be perfect wives, mothers, professionals, and friends, often forgetting to take a moment to appreciate the beauty of the passing years. However, the key to aging gracefully lies not in resisting the passage of time but in accepting it wholeheartedly.

Accepting the passage of time is not about surrendering to the inevitable signs of aging, but rather about embracing the wisdom and experiences that come with it. It is about recognizing that each wrinkle, each grey hair, is a testament to a life well-lived. It is about celebrating the journey we have undertaken and the woman we have become.

As we embark on this journey of accepting the passage of time, we must first cultivate a positive mindset. Society bombards us with unrealistic standards of beauty and youth, leading us to believe that growing older is some

thing to be feared or hidden. However, it is essential to shift our perspective and understand that beauty lies in the diversity of age. Embrace the lines on your face, for they tell a story of resilience, laughter, and love.

To truly embrace the years ahead, it is crucial to prioritize self-care. Nourish your body with wholesome foods, indulge in regular exercise, and pamper yourself with skincare routines that enhance your natural beauty. By taking care of ourselves, we not only improve our physical well-being but also cultivate a sense of self-love that radiates from within.

Furthermore, accepting the passage of time requires us to let go of societal expectations and embrace our individuality. Each one of us has a unique journey, and comparing ourselves to others only hinders our ability to appreciate our growth. Instead, focus on your accomplishments, your dreams, and the joy that each day brings. Embrace the freedom to be exactly who you are, unapologetically.

In conclusion, the art of aging with elegance lies in accepting the passage of time. By shifting our mindset, prioritizing self-care, and embracing our individuality, we can gracefully navigate the years ahead. Remember, dear women, that every day is a gift, and every moment is an opportunity to live authentically and embrace the beauty of each passing year.

CELEBRATING MILESTONES

As women, we are constantly evolving and growing with each passing year. Our lives are filled with countless milestones that shape us into the strong and elegant individuals we are today. In this subchapter, "Celebrating Milestones," we will explore the importance of embracing these milestones and how they contribute to our journey of aging with grace.

Milestones come in all shapes and sizes – from personal achievements to societal milestones. They mark significant moments in our lives, such as graduations, promotions, marriages, the birth of a child, or even the simple act of conquering fear. Each milestone holds a unique significance and deserves to be celebrated.

Celebrating these milestones is not just about throwing a party or receiving gifts. It is about taking the time to acknowledge and honor the growth, resilience, and wisdom that these milestones represent. It is about recognizing the strength within us that has allowed us to overcome obstacles and embrace new opportunities.

By celebrating our milestones, we inspire other women to do the same. Our stories become a source of encouragement and motivation for those who may be facing similar challenges. We show them that aging is not a limitation but a privilege and that each milestone we reach is a testament to our strength and resilience.

Furthermore, celebrating milestones is an opportunity for self-reflection and gratitude. It allows us to pause and appreciate the journey we have taken thus far, acknowledging the lessons we have learned and the person we have become. It reminds us of our ability to adapt and grow, even in the face of adversity.

As we age, celebrating milestones becomes even more vital. It reminds us that aging is not a process of decline, but a continuous journey of self-discovery and personal growth. It encourages us to embrace the changes that come with age, such as wisdom, confidence, and a deeper understanding of ourselves.

In conclusion, "Celebrating Milestones" is a subchapter dedicated to the importance of honoring and embracing the significant moments in our lives. By recognizing and celebrating our milestones, we inspire others, foster gratitude, and uplift ourselves as we age gracefully. Let us celebrate our accomplishments, big and small, and continue to write the beautiful chapters of our lives with elegance and grace.

FINDING PURPOSE
IN EVERY STAGE

As women, our lives are a journey filled with different stages and transitions. From youthful exuberance to the wisdom that comes with age, each phase brings its unique challenges and blessings. It is during these times that we need to find purpose and meaning to truly embrace the beauty of aging with elegance.

In every stage of life, we have the opportunity to find our purpose. Whether we are in our twenties, thirties, forties, or beyond, it is never too late to discover what truly fulfills us. Purpose gives us a reason to wake up each morning, face the day with joy and enthusiasm, and make a difference in the world around us.

Finding purpose in every stage requires self-reflection and a deep understanding of our passions, values, and talents. It is a journey of self-discovery that may take time, but the rewards are immeasurable. By identifying our purpose, we can align our actions and decisions with our true selves, leading to a greater sense of fulfillment and contentment.

In our twenties, we may be focused on building our careers or exploring our passions. Finding purpose during this stage involves taking risks, embracing growth opportunities, and discovering what truly brings us joy. It is a time to nurture our dreams and lay the foundation for our future.

As we move into our thirties and forties, our focus may shift to family, relationships, and personal growth. Our purpose may involve nurturing our loved ones, finding balance in our lives, and making a positive impact on our communities. It is a time to redefine our priorities and find fulfillment in the various roles we play.

As we enter the later stages of life, finding purpose takes on a new dimension. It may involve leaving a legacy, mentoring others, or pursuing lifelong passions that were put on hold. It is a time to embrace the wisdom and experiences we have gained over the years and share them with others.

No matter what stage of life we are in, finding purpose is essential to age with elegance. It gives us a sense of direction and fulfillment that transcends age and allows us to make the most of each day. So, let us embrace the journey of finding purpose in every stage and inspire other women to do the same. For it is through purpose that we can truly age gracefully and embrace the years with elegance.

NURTURING SELF-LOVE
AND SELF-CARE

In the journey of aging gracefully, one of the most vital aspects is nurturing self-love and self-care. As women, we often tend to prioritize the needs of others before our own, forgetting that taking care of ourselves is equally important. In this subchapter, we will explore the significance of self-love and self-care, and how embracing these practices can empower us to navigate the aging process with elegance and positivity.

Self-love is the foundation upon which our overall well-being is built. It involves recognizing our worth, accepting ourselves as we are, and treating ourselves with kindness and compassion. As we age, it becomes even more crucial to cultivate self-love, as society often bombards us with messages that challenge our sense of self-worth. Embracing self-love allows us to celebrate our unique qualities, embrace our years, and live authentically.

Self-care is the act of intentionally nourishing our physical, emotional, and spiritual needs. It encompasses various practices that help us rejuvenate, restore, and

maintain our overall well-being. Incorporating self-care into our daily routines is essential for women as we age. It allows us to prioritize our health and happiness, ensuring that we have the energy and vitality to embrace life's adventures.

Discovering self-love and self-care begins with embracing our changing bodies and appearance. Our bodies are a testament to the incredible journeys we have embarked upon, and they deserve our love and respect. By understanding that beauty comes in all shapes, sizes, and ages, we can let go of societal expectations and celebrate our unique beauty at every stage of life.

Cultivating self-love and self-care also involves setting healthy boundaries and learning to say "no" when necessary. As women, we often find ourselves juggling multiple roles and responsibilities, leaving little time for ourselves. However, by valuing our time and energy, we can create space for self-care activities that replenish our spirits and nurture our well-being.

Furthermore, engaging in activities that bring us joy, such as pursuing hobbies, connecting with loved ones, or exploring new interests, is an essential part of self-love and self-care. These activities allow us to tap into our passions, foster meaningful connections, and create a sense of fulfillment and purpose in our lives.

In conclusion, nurturing self-love and self-care is an integral part of aging with elegance. By prioritizing our own needs, we can embrace our years with grace and positivity. Through self-love, we recognize our worth and celebrate our unique beauty at every stage of life. By practicing self-care, we replenish our spirits, maintain our well-being, and ensure that we have the vitality to navigate life's journey. So, let us embark on this empowering journey of self-love and self-care, embracing our years and inspiring others to do the same.

PRIORITIZING PHYSICAL HEALTH

In the journey of aging gracefully, women need to focus on their physical health. As we embrace the years, it becomes even more crucial to take care of our bodies to maintain a vibrant and fulfilling lifestyle. Prioritizing physical health not only enhances our overall well-being but also allows us to age with elegance and grace. This subchapter will provide valuable insights and practical tips to inspire women in their quest to prioritize their physical health.

1. Understanding the Importance:
Physical health forms the foundation of a happy and fulfilling life. It enables us to carry out daily activities with ease, maintain mental clarity, and enjoy our relationships. By prioritizing physical health, we can prevent chronic diseases, maintain a healthy weight, and increase our energy levels.

2. Incorporating Healthy Habits:
To age gracefully, it's crucial to adopt healthy habits. Regular exercise, such as walking, yoga, or swimming,

helps maintain flexibility, strength, and balance. Engaging in activities we enjoy not only keeps us physically fit but also boosts our mood and reduces stress. Additionally, a balanced diet rich in fruits, vegetables, lean proteins, and whole grains provides the necessary nutrients to support our bodies.

3. Staying Active and Engaged:

As we age, it's important to continue staying active both physically and mentally. Engaging in hobbies, joining social groups, or pursuing volunteer work can help keep our minds sharp and ward off feelings of loneliness or isolation. Regular social interactions and mental stimulation contribute to a sense of purpose and overall well-being.

4. Prioritizing Rest and Self-Care:

While physical activity is essential, it's equally important to prioritize rest and self-care. Adequate sleep and relaxation are vital for the body to rejuvenate and repair itself. Taking time for ourselves, indulging in activities we love, and practicing self-compassion contribute to overall well-being and a positive mindset.

5. Seeking Medical Support:

Regular check-ups and screenings are crucial for maintaining optimal physical health. Consultation with healthcare professionals can help address any concerns or changes in our bodies. Seeking medical support and

advice ensures early detection and effective management of any health issues.

By prioritizing physical health, women can unlock the potential for an elegant and fulfilling aging journey. Embracing regular exercise, adopting healthy habits, staying active and engaged, prioritizing rest and self-care, and seeking medical support are all essential components of aging gracefully. Remember, it's never too late to start prioritizing your physical health. Let this be a reminder to invest in yourself, embrace your years, and live life to the fullest!

CULTIVATING EMOTIONAL WELL-BEING

In the journey of aging gracefully, emotional well-being plays a crucial role in ensuring a fulfilling and joyful life. As women, we face unique challenges as we navigate through the different stages of life. However, by embracing our years and focusing on our emotional well-being, we can cultivate a positive mindset and enhance our overall quality of life.

One of the key aspects of cultivating emotional well-being is self-care. Taking the time to nurture ourselves physically, mentally, and emotionally is essential. This can include engaging in activities that bring us joy, such as hobbies, spending time with loved ones, or pursuing new interests. Prioritizing self-care allows us to recharge, reduce stress, and maintain a healthy balance in our lives.

Another essential element of emotional well-being is fostering strong social connections. As we age, it is vital to

surround ourselves with a supportive network of friends and loved ones. Building and maintaining meaningful relationships can provide us with a sense of belonging, support, and companionship. Whether it's joining community groups, volunteering, or participating in social activities, connecting with others helps combat feelings of isolation and promotes emotional well-being.

Additionally, practicing gratitude and cultivating a positive mindset can have a profound impact on our emotional well-being. By focusing on the present moment and appreciating the blessings in our lives, we can shift our perspective and find joy in even the smallest of things. Incorporating gratitude practices, such as keeping a gratitude journal or expressing appreciation to others, can help us cultivate a positive outlook and enhance our emotional well-being. **Thank God for creating you.**

Furthermore, embracing change and adapting to new circumstances is crucial in the aging process. As we grow older, we may face various life transitions, such as retirement, loss of loved ones, or changes in health. By embracing these changes and seeking opportunities for personal growth, we can navigate these challenges with resilience and grace. Embracing change allows us to focus on the present and embrace new chapters in our lives, fostering emotional well-being.

In conclusion, cultivating emotional well-being is a vital aspect of aging gracefully. By prioritizing self-care, fostering strong social connections, practicing gratitude, and embracing change, we can enhance our emotional well-being and lead fulfilling lives. As women, it is essential to recognize the importance of emotional well-being and make it a priority in our journey of aging with elegance.

Enhancing Spiritual Connection

As women embrace their years and navigate the journey of aging, it becomes increasingly important to nurture and enhance their spiritual connection. In this subchapter, we will explore various practices and perspectives that can help women age gracefully while deepening their spiritual connection.

Spirituality is a deeply personal and individual experience, and it can take many forms. It is a way of finding meaning and purpose in life, connecting with something larger than ourselves, and embracing a sense of inner peace and tranquility. By enhancing our spiritual connection, we can find solace and guidance, even during the challenges that come with aging.

One powerful way to enhance spiritual connection is through mindfulness and meditation practices. These

practices allow women to cultivate a deep sense of presence, quiet the mind, and tune into their inner wisdom. By praying and practicing mindfulness regularly, women can find a sense of peace and clarity that transcends the worries and stresses of daily life.

Another avenue for enhancing spiritual connection is through engaging in acts of kindness and service. As women age, they often find themselves with more time and wisdom to share. By giving back to their communities or volunteering for causes close to their hearts, women can experience a profound sense of purpose and fulfillment.

Exploring and embracing one's own beliefs and values is also an essential aspect of enhancing spiritual connection. This may involve delving deeper into a specific religious or philosophical tradition, or it could mean exploring various spiritual practices and finding what resonates most with one's unique path. The key is to remain open to different perspectives, allowing for personal growth and the deepening of spiritual connection.

Lastly, connecting with nature can be a powerful way for women to enhance their spiritual connection. Spending time in natural surroundings, whether it be walking in a park, gardening, or simply sitting by a window and observing the beauty of the natural world, can bring a sense of awe and wonder. This connection to nature can

help women feel grounded, connected, and in tune with something greater than themselves.

In conclusion, as women age gracefully, nurturing and enhancing their spiritual connection becomes an important aspect of their lives. Through practices such as mindfulness, acts of kindness, exploring personal beliefs, and connecting with nature, women can deepen their spiritual connection, finding solace, meaning, and purpose on their journey of aging with elegance.

CHAPTER 2: CULTIVATING INNER STRENGTH

Developing a Positive Mindset

In the journey of aging gracefully, one of the most powerful tools at a woman's disposal is a positive mindset. It can make all the difference in how she embraces her years and navigates the challenges that come along. A positive mindset is not only about seeing the glass half full, but it is also about cultivating resilience, self-acceptance, and a deep sense of gratitude for the experiences that life brings.

Resilience is at the core of a positive mindset. As women age, they may face physical, emotional, and societal changes that can be overwhelming. However, having a resilient mindset empowers women to bounce back from setbacks and adapt to new circumstances with grace and strength. It allows them to embrace the wisdom that

comes with age and view challenges as opportunities for growth.

Self-acceptance is another crucial aspect of developing a positive mindset. It involves embracing one's flaws and imperfections, and understanding that they are an integral part of who they are. Aging gracefully means accepting the changes that come with time, both externally and internally. By cultivating self-acceptance, women can let go of societal expectations and focus on their unique journey. They can celebrate their accomplishments and acknowledge their worth, regardless of age.

Gratitude is a powerful mindset that can transform every aspect of a woman's life. By practicing gratitude, women can shift their focus from what they lack to what they have. It allows them to appreciate the beauty in small moments, the love of family and friends, and the lessons learned throughout their lives. Gratitude also fosters a sense of contentment and helps women find joy in the present moment.

Developing a positive mindset requires conscious effort and practice. It involves cultivating resilience, practicing self-acceptance, and embracing gratitude. Surrounding oneself with positive influences, such as supportive friends and uplifting literature, can greatly aid in this journey. Additionally, engaging in activities that bring joy and fulfillment, such as hobbies, volunteering, or

pursuing personal interests, can further enhance a positive mindset.

By developing a positive mindset, women can truly age with elegance. They can navigate the challenges that come with aging gracefully, finding strength in resilience, self-acceptance, and gratitude. A positive mindset empowers women to embrace their years, celebrate their unique journeys, and inspire others to do the same. Remember, age is just a number, and with a positive mindset, the possibilities for growth and fulfillment are endless.

SHIFTING PERSPECTIVES ON AGING

In today's society, the perception of aging has undergone a remarkable transformation. Gone are the days when women were expected to hide their years and feel ashamed of growing older. Instead, a new movement has emerged—one that encourages women to embrace the beauty and wisdom that come with age. This subchapter, titled "Shifting Perspectives on Aging," aims to inspire women to age gracefully and celebrate the various stages of life.

Throughout history, aging has often been associated with negative connotations. Women were expected to adhere to societal standards of youth and beauty, fearing the natural process of getting older. However, in recent years, there has been a powerful shift in attitudes towards aging. Women have started to recognize that age brings a wealth of experiences, knowledge, and self-assurance that cannot be found in youth alone.

This subchapter delves into the various aspects of this shifting perspective on aging. It delves into the importance of self-care and maintaining a positive mindset as women navigate the different stages of life. It emphasizes the significance of embracing one's physical appearance and finding confidence in the unique beauty that comes with age.

Moreover, this subchapter explores the idea of aging as a journey of self-discovery and personal growth. It encourages women to use their years to explore new passions, pursue long-held dreams, and redefine their purpose. It highlights the stories of inspiring women who have defied societal expectations and achieved remarkable success in their later years.

Additionally, this subchapter discusses the importance of community and support networks for women as they age. It emphasizes the power of female friendships and the role they play in fostering a sense of belonging and empowerment. It also provides practical advice on finding support systems and creating a fulfilling social life during the later stages of life.

By the end of this subchapter, readers will be equipped with a renewed perspective on aging—one that embraces the elegance and beauty that comes with growing older. They will be inspired to celebrate their years and view aging as an opportunity for self-discovery, personal

growth, and making a positive impact on the world. Through embracing their years, these women will find the strength and confidence to age gracefully and inspire others to do the same.

PRACTICING GRATITUDE AND MINDFULNESS

In the journey of aging gracefully, one powerful tool that can transform our perception of life's challenges and bring about a sense of inner peace is the practice of gratitude and mindfulness. As women, we often find ourselves juggling multiple roles, dealing with societal expectations, and navigating the physical and emotional changes that come with age. However, by incorporating gratitude and mindfulness into our daily lives, we can embrace our years with elegance and find joy in the present moment.

Gratitude, often described as the attitude of appreciation, has the power to shift our focus from what is lacking in our lives to what we already have. It invites us to acknowledge and cherish the blessings, both big and small, that surround us every day. By cultivating a grateful mindset, we can counteract the negative thoughts and anxieties that may arise as we age. The simple act of expressing gratitude for our health, relationships, ex

periences, and even the challenges we have overcome, can create a ripple effect of positivity and contentment in our lives.

Mindfulness, on the other hand, is about being fully present in the moment, without judgment or attachment. It encourages us to observe our thoughts, emotions, and sensations with curiosity and acceptance. As women on the journey of aging, mindfulness can help us navigate the changes in our bodies and emotions with grace and self-compassion. By practicing mindfulness, we can learn to embrace the inevitable transitions of life with equanimity, whether it's the physical changes in our appearance or the emotional adjustments that come with transitioning into different life stages.

Together, gratitude and mindfulness form a powerful duo that can help us find joy and purpose in our everyday lives. By incorporating gratitude practices such as keeping a gratitude journal, expressing appreciation to loved ones, or simply taking a moment each day to reflect on what we are grateful for, we can cultivate a resilient and positive mindset. Additionally, integrating mindfulness into our routines through practices like meditation, deep breathing, or mindful movement can enhance our ability to stay present and grounded as we navigate the challenges and joys of aging.

In conclusion, embracing gratitude and mindfulness can empower women to age with elegance and grace. By adopting a grateful mindset and practicing mindfulness, we can transform our perspective on aging, finding beauty and fulfillment in each passing year. Let us embark on this journey together, supporting and inspiring one another to live our lives with gratitude, presence, and the wisdom that comes with embracing our years.

OVERCOMING SELF-LIMITING BELIEFS

In the journey of aging gracefully, one of the biggest obstacles we often face is our own self-limiting beliefs. These beliefs can hold us back from embracing all that life has to offer and prevent us from truly enjoying our years. However, it is never too late to challenge these beliefs and cultivate a mindset of empowerment and possibility.

As women, we have been conditioned by society to believe that aging is synonymous with decline and loss. We are bombarded with messages that tell us we are no longer attractive or relevant as we grow older. These negative beliefs can seep into our subconscious and become deeply ingrained, holding us back from fully embracing the beauty and wisdom that comes with age.

But it is time for a shift in perspective. It is time for us to break free from these self-imposed limitations and redefine what it means to age with elegance. We must recognize that our worth is not determined by our physical appearance or societal standards, but rather by the

strength, resilience, and wisdom we have gained over the years.

Overcoming self-limiting beliefs begins with self-awareness. Take the time to examine the beliefs that may be holding you back. Are you telling yourself that you are too old to pursue new passions or start a new career? Are you allowing fear of judgment to prevent you from taking risks and trying new things? Recognize that these beliefs are not based on truth, but rather on societal conditioning.

Once you have identified these self-limiting beliefs, it is important to challenge them head-on. Surround yourself with positive influences and role models who defy age stereotypes. Seek out empowering literature, and attend workshops or seminars that promote self-acceptance and personal growth. Surround yourself with a supportive network of women who uplift and inspire you.

Remember, aging with elegance is about embracing all aspects of ourselves and living our lives to the fullest. It is about redefining what it means to be a woman of a certain age and celebrating the wisdom and experience that comes with it. Let go of self-limiting beliefs and open yourself up to the endless possibilities that await you. Embrace your years with grace and confidence, knowing that you are a force to be reckoned with at any age.

BUILDING RESILIENCE AND ADAPTABILITY

In our journey through life, we encounter numerous challenges and changes that can test our strength and ability to adapt. As women, we have the unique opportunity to age gracefully, embracing each passing year with elegance and grace. To navigate this path successfully, it is crucial to build resilience and adaptability within ourselves.

Resilience is the capacity to bounce back from adversity, to remain strong and optimistic in the face of challenges. It is a quality that can be cultivated, allowing us to not only survive but thrive during difficult times. By building resilience, we can weather the storms of life while still maintaining our sense of self-worth and purpose.

To develop resilience, it is crucial to cultivate a positive mindset. By reframing negative thoughts and focusing on the possibilities that lie ahead, we can build a strong mental foundation. Surrounding ourselves with supportive and positive people is also key, as their encour

agement and love can help us stay resilient in the face of adversity.

Adaptability, on the other hand, is the ability to adjust and acclimate to new circumstances or changes in our lives. As we age, our bodies and minds undergo transformations that require us to adapt and find new ways of doing things. Embracing change and being open to new experiences is essential for maintaining a sense of vitality and zest for life.

One of the best ways to foster adaptability is by challenging ourselves to step outside our comfort zones. Trying new activities, learning new skills, and exploring different hobbies can help us stay mentally agile and adaptable. It is also important to maintain a healthy lifestyle, taking care of our physical and emotional well-being. Regular exercise, a balanced diet, and self-care practices can all contribute to our ability to adapt to the changes that come with aging.

Building resilience and adaptability is an ongoing process. It requires a commitment to personal growth and a willingness to embrace the challenges and changes that come our way. By cultivating these qualities within ourselves, we can age with elegance and inspire others to do the same. Let us embrace our years with grace, knowing that our resilience and adaptability will carry us through every season of life.

EMBRACING CHANGE WITH GRACE

Change is an inevitable part of life. As women, we experience a multitude of changes throughout our lives - from the physical changes that come with aging to the emotional and spiritual transformations that shape us into the remarkable individuals we are today. In the subchapter "Embracing Change with Grace" of the book "Aging with Elegance: Inspiring Women to Embrace Their Years," we delve into the importance of accepting change and navigating it with poise and resilience.

As we age, our bodies undergo a series of transformations. The youthful glow we once possessed may fade, and we may notice wrinkles and gray hairs gradually making their appearance. However, it is crucial to remember that beauty transcends mere physical attributes. Aging gracefully is about embracing these changes and recognizing the wisdom and experiences that come with them. It is about feeling confident and comfortable in our skin, radiating a beauty that stems from within.

Embracing change also means acknowledging the shifting roles and responsibilities we encounter as we move through different stages of life. From the carefree days of youth to the nurturing role of motherhood and the fulfilling roles we undertake in our careers, each phase presents its own set of challenges and rewards. By accepting and adapting to these changes, we can find fulfillment and purpose in every stage of our lives.

Change, however, extends beyond the external and encompasses our emotional and spiritual realms as well. Life's circumstances may throw us off balance, testing our resilience and strength. Embracing change with grace means cultivating a sense of inner peace and learning to navigate through life's ups and downs with resilience and positivity. It is about finding the silver linings in every situation and harnessing the power of gratitude to transform challenges into opportunities for growth.

To help women age gracefully, it is essential to create a supportive community of like-minded individuals who understand and empathize with our experiences. By fostering relationships with other women who are on a similar journey, we can share stories, insights, and wisdom, providing mutual support and encouragement.

In conclusion, "Embracing Change with Grace" is an invitation to women to celebrate the beauty and strength that comes with age. It encourages us to embrace the

physical, emotional, and spiritual changes that life presents and navigate through them with elegance and resilience. Through acceptance, gratitude, and a supportive community, we can truly age with elegance and inspire others to do the same.

LEARNING FROM LIFE'S CHALLENGES

Life is an intricate tapestry of experiences, filled with both triumphs and challenges. As women, we have encountered numerous obstacles throughout our journey, but it is in these moments of adversity that we have the opportunity to grow, learn, and ultimately, age with elegance. In this subchapter, titled "Learning from Life's Challenges," we will explore how these hardships can serve as valuable lessons, empowering us to embrace our years with grace and wisdom.

One of the most significant aspects of learning from life's challenges is developing resilience. Resilience allows us to bounce back from difficult situations, enabling us to navigate the changing landscape of aging with grace and strength. By facing and overcoming challenging circumstances, we become more resilient, acquiring the tools necessary to cope with future obstacles. Through the stories of inspiring women who have gracefully aged despite adversities, we will learn how to cultivate resilience in our own lives.

Moreover, life's challenges provide us with unique opportunities for personal growth and self-discovery. They allow us to uncover hidden strengths and talents that may have otherwise remained dormant. By embracing these challenges, we can unlock our full potential and find new passions and purpose in our lives, regardless of age. We will explore stories of women who have reinvented themselves in the face of adversity, proving that it is never too late to pursue our dreams and aspirations.

Additionally, learning from life's challenges helps us cultivate empathy and compassion for others. Through our own experiences of overcoming obstacles, we gain a deeper understanding of the struggles faced by those around us. This newfound empathy allows us to support and uplift other women as they navigate their unique journeys. We will discuss the importance of building strong connections with other women and the power of sharing our stories to inspire and encourage one another.

In conclusion, the subchapter "Learning from Life's Challenges" serves as a guide to help women age gracefully by embracing the lessons that come from adversity. By developing resilience, uncovering hidden strengths, and cultivating empathy, we can navigate the complexities of aging with elegance. Through the stories of inspiring women, we will learn that life's challenges are not obstacles to be feared but opportunities for growth, trans

formation, and ultimately, embracing our years with grace and wisdom.

DISCOVERING HIDDEN STRENGTHS

Subchapter: Discovering Hidden Strengths

Introduction:
As women, we often find ourselves fixated on the external aspects of aging - the wrinkles, gray hair, and the physical changes that come with the passing years. However, in the journey of aging gracefully, it is equally important to explore the hidden strengths that lie within us. These hidden strengths are the pillars that can support us through life's challenges and empower us to embrace our years with elegance. In this subchapter, we delve into the process of discovering these hidden strengths and how they can help women age gracefully.

Unleashing Your Inner Resilience:
Resilience is a remarkable strength that women possess, enabling us to bounce back from adversity. It is import

ant to recognize this inherent resilience within ourselves and understand how it can be harnessed as we age. By embracing life's ups and downs, learning from setbacks, and cultivating a positive mindset, we can tap into our inner resilience and navigate the challenges that come with aging.

Embracing Wisdom and Experiences:
One of the most valuable hidden strengths that age brings is the accumulation of wisdom and experiences. Each chapter of life has taught us valuable lessons and shaped us into the women we are today. By embracing these experiences and sharing our wisdom with others, we not only enrich our own lives but also inspire and uplift those around us. Aging gracefully means recognizing the power of our experiences and using them to guide and support others.

Cultivating Self-Compassion:
As women, we often tend to be hard on ourselves, especially as we age. However, practicing self-compassion is a powerful hidden strength that can transform our journey. By treating ourselves with kindness, understanding, and forgiveness, we can embrace our imperfections and focus on self-growth. Cultivating self-compassion allows us to accept ourselves as we are and find joy in the process of aging.

Nurturing Relationships:
Our relationships, both old and new, are a source of immense strength as we age. Nurturing these connections, be it with family, friends, or communities, can provide us with a sense of belonging, support, and purpose. By
investing time and effort into building and maintaining meaningful relationships, we can create a strong support system that helps us age gracefully.

Conclusion:

Discovering our hidden strengths is an essential part of aging with elegance. By unleashing our resilience, embracing our wisdom, cultivating self-compassion, and nurturing relationships, we can navigate the journey of aging gracefully. As women, we have a wealth of inner resources waiting to be explored and celebrated. Let us embark on this empowering journey together, embracing our hidden strengths and inspiring others to do the same.

CHAPTER 3: NURTURING RELATIONSHIPS AND CONNECTIONS

Embracing Connection with Others

In the journey of aging gracefully, one of the most vital aspects is enabling and nurturing connections with others. As women, we have a natural inclination towards socializing and building relationships, and these connections can play a significant role in enhancing our overall well-being and happiness as we age.

As we gracefully embrace our years, it is crucial to recognize the power and importance of surrounding ourselves with a supportive and loving community. Building and maintaining connections with others can provide us with a sense of belonging, purpose, and fulfillment.

First and foremost, let us celebrate the friendships we have cultivated over the years. Our friends are the pillars of strength who have stood by us through thick and thin. They provide invaluable emotional support, laughter, and companionship. By cherishing and investing in these relationships, we create a nurturing environment that enriches our lives and helps us navigate the challenges that come with aging.

However, it is equally important to seek out new connections and embrace new experiences. Expanding our social circles allows us to meet like-minded individuals who can bring fresh perspectives and enrich our lives. Whether it's joining a book club, attending community events, or participating in volunteer work, these activities can introduce us to new friends and opportunities for personal growth.

In today's digital age, technology can also play a significant role in fostering connections. Social media platforms, online forums, and video chat applications can help us stay connected with loved ones who may be physically distant. Embracing technology allows us to bridge the gap and maintain meaningful relationships, even when face-to-face interactions are not possible.

Moreover, nurturing connections with younger generations can bring a renewed sense of purpose and joy into our lives. By sharing our wisdom, experiences, and

stories, we can inspire and empower the next generation of women. Mentoring programs, intergenerational activities, and volunteering with youth organizations are fantastic ways to foster these connections and leave a lasting impact.

In conclusion, embracing connection with others is an essential aspect of aging with elegance. By nurturing existing relationships, seeking out new connections, leveraging technology, and fostering intergenerational bonds, we can build a strong support system that enhances our well-being and allows us to age gracefully. Remember, it is through these connections that we find strength, love, and joy on our journey.

Building and Maintaining Friendships

Friendships play a crucial role in our lives, regardless of age. As women, we understand the value and importance of having strong and supportive relationships. As we age, it becomes even more crucial to cultivate and maintain these friendships to help us navigate the ups and downs of life with grace and elegance.

One of the key aspects of building and maintaining friendships as we age is embracing authenticity. It is essential to be true to ourselves and allow our vulnerability to shine through. By being authentic, we attract like-

minded individuals who appreciate us for who we are, our flaws and all. Surrounding ourselves with genuine friends who accept us unconditionally can immensely contribute to our overall well-being.

Another vital aspect of building and maintaining friendships is investing time and effort. As we age, life tends to get busier with various responsibilities, such as career and family. However, it is crucial to prioritize our friendships and make time for them. Regularly checking in with our friends through phone calls, coffee dates, or even virtual meet-ups can help foster a deeper connection and ensure that our friendships continue to grow.

Moreover, it is important to be a good listener and offer support to our friends. As we age, we face unique challenges, such as health issues or loss of loved ones. Being there for our friends during their difficult times can strengthen our bond and provide them with the comfort they need. By actively listening without judgment and offering a shoulder to lean on, we can create a safe space for our friends to share their joys and struggles.

Additionally, embracing new experiences and expanding our social circles can help us build new friendships as we age. Joining clubs, attending social events, or volunteering for causes we are passionate about can introduce us to like-minded individuals and potential lifelong friends.

It is never too late to make new connections and enrich our lives with new friendships.

In conclusion, as women, it is important for us to recognize the significance of building and maintaining friendships as we age gracefully. By embracing authenticity, investing time and effort, being a good listener, and embracing new experiences, we can cultivate strong and supportive friendships that will accompany us through the journey of aging with elegance. Let us cherish and nurture our friendships, for they are the invaluable treasures that make our lives truly fulfilling.

Strengthening Family Bonds

In the journey of aging gracefully, one of the most valuable and fulfilling aspects of life is the bond we share with our family. Our loved ones provide us with the support, love, and sense of belonging that can make the aging process more enjoyable and meaningful. Strengthening these family bonds is an essential part of embracing our years and living with elegance.

As women, we often take on the role of the caregiver, nurturing and supporting our families throughout our lives. However, as we age, it becomes crucial to prioritize our well-being while also nurturing these relationships. By investing time and effort in strengthening family

bonds, we can create a loving and supportive environment that benefits both ourselves and our loved ones.

One way to strengthen family bonds is through open and honest communication. As we age, we may have different needs and expectations, and it is important to express these to our family members. By openly discussing our desires, concerns, and dreams, we can foster understanding and create a deeper connection with our loved ones. This communication should be a two-way street, allowing us to listen to the thoughts and feelings of our family members as well.

Creating shared experiences and traditions is another powerful way to strengthen family bonds. Whether it's gathering for a weekly family dinner, taking annual vacations together, or engaging in hobbies and activities as a group, these shared moments can create lasting memories and a sense of unity. By intentionally carving out time for these activities, we can build stronger connections with our family members and create a support system that will be there for us as we age.

Furthermore, it is important to acknowledge and celebrate the individuality of each family member. As we age, it becomes even more significant to respect and appreciate the unique qualities and contributions of our loved ones. By fostering an environment of acceptance and support, we can ensure that everyone feels valued

and loved, strengthening the bonds that hold our family together.

In conclusion, strengthening family bonds is an integral part of aging gracefully. By prioritizing open communication, creating shared experiences, and celebrating individuality, we can cultivate a loving and supportive environment that enriches our lives and the lives of our loved ones. Embracing and nurturing these connections will not only help us age with elegance but also provide a strong foundation of love and support as we navigate the journey of life.

Embracing Intergenerational Relationships

In the journey of aging gracefully, one of the most valuable and enriching experiences a woman can have is developing intergenerational relationships. These connections with younger generations not only provide a sense of purpose and fulfillment but also offer unique opportunities for personal growth, learning, and mutual support.

As women, we often find ourselves surrounded by the wisdom and experiences of those who came before us. However, it is equally important to recognize the value of bridging the generation gap and embracing the perspectives and ideas of younger women. By fostering inter

generational relationships, we create a space for mutual understanding, empathy, and shared wisdom.

One of the most significant benefits of intergenerational relationships is the opportunity to learn from each other. Younger women bring fresh perspectives, technological savvy, and new approaches to life's challenges. By engaging with them, we can broaden our horizons, stay current with the ever-changing world, and continue to grow intellectually and emotionally. Likewise, our years of experience and accumulated wisdom can offer valuable guidance, mentorship, and a sense of grounding to younger generations.

Moreover, intergenerational relationships provide a vital support system for women of all ages. The shared experiences, stories, and understanding that come from these connections create a sense of belonging and community. Whether it is through formal mentorship programs, volunteering, or simply building friendships with younger women, these relationships can be a source of inspiration, encouragement, and emotional support throughout the aging process.

Embracing intergenerational relationships also offers an opportunity to leave a lasting legacy. By sharing our stories, life lessons, and personal values with younger women, we contribute to the preservation and transmission of our collective wisdom. In turn, this knowledge

can empower future generations of women to navigate the challenges of aging with grace, resilience, and confidence.

In conclusion, embracing intergenerational relationships is a powerful way for women to age with elegance. By cultivating connections with younger generations, we open ourselves up to a world of learning, support, and personal growth. These relationships not only enrich our lives but also allow us to leave a lasting impact on the lives of those who will follow in our footsteps. Let us embrace the beauty of intergenerational connections and inspire each other to embrace our years with grace, wisdom, and a sense of purpose.

Exploring New Opportunities for Social Engagement

As women, we have always been the backbone of our families, communities, and society. As we age gracefully, we need to continue nurturing our social connections and exploring new opportunities for social engagement. By doing so, we not only enhance our well-being but also contribute to the betterment of those around us.

Social engagement plays a vital role in helping women age with elegance. It provides a platform for us to connect with like-minded individuals, share experiences,

and find support in our journey through life. By actively participating in social activities, we can cultivate a sense of belonging, boost our self-esteem, and maintain a positive outlook on aging.

One way to explore new opportunities for social engagement is by joining community organizations or clubs that align with our interests or passions. Whether it be a book club, a gardening society, or a volunteer group, these organizations provide a space for us to meet new people, exchange ideas, and contribute to causes close to our hearts. Engaging in such activities not only keeps our minds sharp but also fosters personal growth and fulfillment.

Technology has also opened up a world of possibilities for social engagement. Online communities and social media platforms can connect us with people from all walks of life, regardless of geographical boundaries. We can find forums, groups, and networks dedicated to topics ranging from art and culture to health and wellness. These digital spaces offer a wealth of knowledge, support, and opportunities for meaningful connections.

Furthermore, embracing new opportunities for social engagement can also involve pursuing lifelong learning. Enrolling in classes, workshops, or seminars allows us to expand our horizons, acquire new skills, and meet individuals who share similar interests. The joy of learning

and the camaraderie built through educational experiences can be incredibly fulfilling and enriching.

It is important for us, as women, to recognize the value of social engagement as we age. By actively seeking out new opportunities for connection and interaction, we can continue to grow, learn, and contribute to our communities. So let us embrace the chance to explore new avenues for social engagement, for it is through these experiences that we can truly age with elegance.

Engaging in Community Activities

One of the key aspects of aging gracefully is staying connected and engaged with the world around us. As women, we have a unique opportunity to make a positive impact in our communities, not only for ourselves but also for future generations. Engaging in community activities is not only a way to stay active and involved, but it also allows us to give back and make a difference.

There are countless ways for women to get involved in their communities, no matter their interests or abilities. Volunteering is a great way to start. Whether it's at a local food bank, a hospital, or an animal shelter, there are always organizations in need of helping hands. By giving our time and skills, we can contribute to causes that are close to our hearts and make a tangible difference in the lives of others.

Engaging in community activities also provides an opportunity to learn and grow. Joining a book club, attending workshops or seminars, or even taking up a new hobby can expand our horizons and keep our minds sharp. These activities not only provide intellectual stimulation but also foster new friendships and social connections.

Furthermore, community engagement allows us to share our wisdom and experience with younger generations. By mentoring, teaching, or participating in intergenerational programs, we can inspire and guide younger women, helping them navigate their journeys with grace and resilience.

Engaging in community activities can also be a source of personal fulfillment and happiness. Whether it's participating in local cultural events, starting a community garden, or even organizing a neighborhood clean-up, these activities bring a sense of purpose and meaning to our lives. They remind us that we still have so much to offer and that our contributions are valuable.

As women, we have a unique perspective and a wealth of experience to bring to the table. Embracing community

activities allows us to use our voices and make a positive impact in the world. It is through these engagements that we can continue to grow, learn, and inspire others to age with elegance and grace.

So, let us embrace the opportunities that community involvement brings. Let us step out of our comfort zones, connect with others, and make a difference in our communities. Together, as women, we can create a brighter future for ourselves and those who will come after us.

Volunteering and Giving Back

In the journey of aging gracefully, one aspect that holds great significance is the act of giving back to others. Volunteering not only enriches our lives but also positively impacts those around us. As women navigating the beautiful years of aging, we have a unique opportunity to make a difference in the lives of others as well as our own.

Volunteering allows us to tap into our skills, knowledge, and experiences, empowering us to share our wisdom with the world. It provides a sense of purpose, fulfillment, and renewed passion for life. By engaging in meaningful activities that help others, we can find new avenues for personal growth and self-discovery.

There are countless ways for women to embrace the spirit of giving back. One option is to become involved with organizations that support and empower women. By volunteering at women's shelters, mentoring programs, or organizations that provide resources for women in need, we can have a direct impact on their lives. Sharing our own stories and experiences can serve as a source of inspiration and encouragement for those who may be facing similar challenges.

Another avenue is to extend a helping hand to the elderly in our communities. Many senior citizens experience loneliness and isolation, and a simple act of kindness can brighten their day. Volunteering at local senior centers or organizing social events can foster a sense of community and companionship, while also creating cherished memories.

Furthermore, we can contribute to causes that align with our passions and interests. Whether it is environmental conservation, animal welfare, or education, numerous organizations rely on volunteers. By offering our time and skills, we can actively participate in creating a better world for future generations.

Volunteering also provides an opportunity for personal growth and learning. It allows us to step outside our comfort zones, acquire new skills, and build meaningful connections with like-minded individuals. The sense

of fulfillment and purpose gained from giving back can greatly enhance our overall well-being.

As women, we possess an incredible capacity for empathy, compassion, and understanding. By embracing the spirit of volunteering and giving back, we can leave a lasting impact on the lives of others, while also enriching our own. Let us seize this opportunity to make a difference, inspire change, and age with elegance. Together, we can create a world where women of all ages are empowered, cherished, and celebrated.

Joining Supportive Networks

One of the key aspects of aging gracefully is building a strong support system. As women, we often find solace in connecting with others who are going through similar experiences and challenges. Joining supportive networks can provide us with a sense of belonging, understanding, and empowerment as we navigate the journey of aging.

Supportive networks can take various forms, ranging from social clubs and organizations to online communities and support groups. These networks offer a safe space where women can share their thoughts, concerns, and triumphs with like-minded individuals. By joining these networks, we can forge new friendships, gain valu

able insights, and find comfort in knowing that we are not alone.

One of the benefits of joining supportive networks is the opportunity to exchange knowledge and learn from one another. Women who have already experienced the different stages of aging can offer valuable advice and guidance to those who are just starting their journey. Additionally, being part of a supportive network allows us to stay updated on the latest trends, research, and resources related to aging gracefully. This knowledge empowers us to make informed decisions about our health, well-being, and lifestyle choices.

Supportive networks also provide a sense of camaraderie and emotional support. Sharing our joys and sorrows with others who understand our unique challenges can be incredibly therapeutic. These networks create a space where we can freely express our emotions, seek advice, and find comfort during difficult times.

Furthermore, joining supportive networks can lead to opportunities for personal growth and self-discovery. Engaging in activities and discussions with like-minded individuals can spark new interests and passions. These networks often organize workshops, seminars, and events that promote personal development and lifelong learning. By being an active participants, we can broaden

our horizons, discover new talents, and redefine our self-perception as we age.

In conclusion, joining supportive networks is an essential step in embracing our years and aging gracefully. These networks offer us a sense of belonging, empowerment, and emotional support. By connecting with other women who are going through similar experiences, we can gain valuable insights, exchange knowledge, and find comfort in knowing that we are not alone. Furthermore, these networks provide opportunities for personal growth and self-discovery, allowing us to redefine our identity as we navigate the journey of aging. So, let us embrace the power of supportive networks and unlock the potential for an elegant and fulfilling aging experience.

CHAPTER 4: EMBRACING BEAUTY AT ANY AGE

Celebrating Individual Style and Fashion

Subchapter: Celebrating Individual Style and Fashion

Introduction:

In our journey of aging gracefully, it is crucial to recognize and embrace the power of individual style and fashion. As women, we possess a unique ability to express ourselves through what we wear, allowing our personalities to shine and radiate confidence. In this subchapter, we will explore how celebrating our style and fashion choices can enhance our self-esteem, redefine beauty standards, and inspire us to embrace the beauty of our years.

1. Embracing Self-Expression:

Fashion is a form of self-expression that speaks volumes about who we are as individuals. As we age, it becomes even more important to embrace our style, letting go of societal expectations and embracing what truly makes us feel comfortable and beautiful. By celebrating our individuality through fashion, we can proudly showcase our unique personalities and experiences, inspiring others to do the same.

2. Redefining Beauty Standards:

In a world that often promotes youth and perfection as the epitome of beauty, women must redefine these standards. Aging with elegance means embracing our beauty and recognizing the value that comes with experience and wisdom. By celebrating our style, we challenge the notion that beauty is limited to a specific age or body type. We encourage women to embrace their unique features and confidently redefine what it means to be beautiful.

3. Cultivating Confidence:

Our style and fashion choices have the power to boost our self-esteem and cultivate confidence. When we feel good about what we wear, we exude a sense of self-assurance that is contagious. By celebrating our individuality,

we inspire other women to embrace their style and confidently navigate the different phases of life.

4. Embracing the Beauty of Our Years:

Aging gracefully is about embracing the beauty that comes with each passing year. Our style and fashion choices should reflect the confidence and wisdom we have gained throughout our lives. By celebrating our individuality, we encourage other women to embrace their years and cherish the journey they have embarked upon.

Conclusion:

As women, our individual styles and fashion choices play a significant role in how we age gracefully. By celebrating our uniqueness, redefining beauty standards, cultivating confidence, and embracing the beauty of our years, we inspire ourselves and other women to live authentically and confidently. So, let us celebrate our style and fashion, for it is a reflection of our inner strength and elegance.

Dressing Confidently for Every Occasion

Dressing Confidently for Every Occasion: Master the Art of Aging with Elegance

Introduction:
As women, our style evolves with time, just like we do. Embracing our years gracefully means not only taking care of our bodies and minds but also dressing confidently for every occasion. Our clothing choices can be a powerful tool to express our personality, boost our self-esteem, and radiate elegance. In this subchapter, we will explore the secrets of dressing confidently and stylishly, ensuring that every woman can age with grace and poise.

1. Understanding Your Body:

The first step towards dressing confidently is understanding and embracing our unique body shape. We are all beautiful in our way, and by recognizing our body's strengths, we can highlight them with the right clothing choices. From pear-shaped to hourglass figures, we will delve into various body types and provide tailored tips on how to accentuate our best features.

2. Developing a Signature Style:
Creating a signature style that reflects our personal

ity and complements our age is essential for confident dressing. We will explore how to curate a timeless wardrobe, focusing on quality pieces that can be mixed and matched effortlessly. From classic staples to statement accessories, we will guide women in building a collection that exudes elegance and sophistication.

3. Dressing for Different Occasions:
Whether it's a casual outing, a formal event, or a professional meeting, dressing appropriately for each occasion is crucial for feeling confident. We will discuss the dos and don'ts of dressing for various events, offering practical advice on selecting the right attire, colors, and accessories. By mastering the art of dressing for different occasions, women can tackle any event with poise and style.

4. Navigating Trends:
While trends come and go, true elegance remains timeless. We will discuss how to incorporate current fashion trends into our wardrobes without compromising our style. Understanding which trends suit our age, body type, and lifestyle will enable women to stay fashionable while staying true to themselves.

5. Embracing Aging Gracefully:
Aging is a beautiful journey, and our clothing choices

should reflect our wisdom and confidence. We will delve into how to embrace our changing bodies and adapt our style to suit our evolving needs. From embracing comfortable yet stylish fabrics to experimenting with mature makeup looks, we will guide embracing aging gracefully through our fashion choices.

Conclusion:
Dressing confidently for every occasion is an art that every woman can master. By understanding our bodies, developing a signature style, dressing appropriately for different occasions, navigating trends, and embracing aging gracefully, we can truly age with elegance. Let this subchapter be your guide as you embark on a journey of self-expression, self-acceptance, and sartorial confidence. Together, let's inspire women to embrace their years with grace and radiate elegance through their fashion choices.

Adapting Fashion Trends to Personal Taste

Fashion is a powerful tool that allows us to express our personalities, boost our confidence, and make a statement about who we are. As we age, it becomes even more important to adapt fashion trends to our tastes, as it helps us maintain a sense of elegance and individuality. In this subchapter, we will explore the art of embracing fashion trends while staying true to our unique style, helping women age gracefully and confidently.

The first step in adapting to fashion trends is understanding our tastes. It is vital to be aware of our body

type, preferences, and what makes us feel comfortable and

beautiful. This knowledge serves as a foundation for making informed fashion choices. Once we have a clear understanding of our taste, we can confidently explore the ever-changing world of fashion trends.

However, it is important to remember that not all trends are suitable for every woman. That is where the art of adaptation comes into play. Instead of blindly following trends, we can cherry-pick elements that resonate with our style. For instance, if bold patterns are in vogue but don't align with our taste, we can incorporate them through accessories like scarves or handbags, or simply opt for a more subtle interpretation.

Another way to adapt fashion trends is by incorporating them into our existing wardrobe. By mixing and matching new pieces with our classic favorites, we create a unique and timeless style that is truly our own. This approach allows us to stay current without compromising our taste or spending a fortune on a complete wardrobe overhaul.

Furthermore, embracing fashion trends to suit our taste also involves considering our lifestyle and the occasions we dress for. As we age, our social calendar may change, and we might find ourselves attending more formal events or enjoying a more relaxed retirement lifestyle.

Adapting fashion trends to fit these situations ensures we always feel appropriate and confident in our attire.

In conclusion, adapting fashion trends to our taste is a skill that helps women age gracefully and embrace their years with elegance. By understanding our style, selectively incorporating trends, mixing new pieces with classics, and considering our lifestyle, we can confidently navigate the ever-changing fashion world. Remember, fashion is not about conforming but about expressing our unique selves, and by doing so, we can truly age with elegance.

Enhancing Natural Beauty with Makeup

Makeup has long been celebrated as a powerful tool to enhance our natural beauty and boost our confidence. As we age, it becomes even more important to embrace this art form and adapt our techniques to suit our changing features. In this subchapter, we will explore how makeup can help women age gracefully, allowing them to feel beautiful and confident at any stage of life.

First and foremost, it is crucial to understand that makeup should never be used to mask our true selves or hide our age. Instead, it should serve as a means to celebrate our unique features and enhance our natural beauty. By using the right products and techniques, we

can emphasize our best attributes while embracing the wisdom and grace that comes with age.

One of the key aspects of aging gracefully is maintaining healthy and radiant skin. As we grow older, our skin may require extra care and nourishment. With the right skincare routine, including proper cleansing, moisturizing, and protection from the sun, we can create a flawless canvas for our makeup application. Furthermore, incorporating anti-aging products such as serums and creams can help minimize the appearance of fine lines and wrinkles, allowing our makeup to glide on smoothly.

When it comes to makeup application, less is often more. Opting for a lightweight foundation or tinted moisturizer can provide a natural-looking base while allowing our skin to breathe. By using a concealer to target specific areas of concern, such as dark circles or age spots, we can achieve a more youthful and even complexion.

Eyes are said to be the windows to the soul, and they deserve special attention. As we age, our eyelashes may become sparse, and our eyelids may lose their firmness. By using an eyelash curler and mascara, we can instantly open up our eyes and create a more youthful appearance. Additionally, choosing neutral eyeshadow shades and avoiding heavy eyeliner can help to maintain a soft and natural look.

Lastly, our lips deserve some love and care. As we age, our lips may lose their plumpness and definition. By using a lip balm or primer, we can hydrate our lips and prevent the feathering of lipstick. Opting for colors that complement our skin tone and choosing creamy or satin finishes can create a more youthful and luscious pout.

In conclusion, enhancing our natural beauty with makeup is an art form that can help women age gracefully. By embracing our changing features and using the right products and techniques, we can celebrate our unique beauty at every stage of life. Remember, true elegance comes from within, and makeup is simply a tool to enhance the confidence and radiance that shines from within us.

Nurturing a Healthy Body Image

In our society, women are bombarded with unrealistic beauty

standards and messages that suggest growing older is something to be feared or fought against. However, embracing the aging process and taking care of our bodies is essential for leading a fulfilling and confident life. In this subchapter, we will explore strategies to nurture a healthy body image and help women age gracefully.

First and foremost, it is vital to recognize that beauty comes in all shapes, sizes, and ages. Embrace your unique features and celebrate the wisdom and experiences that come with aging. Instead of focusing on societal expectations, shift your mindset towards self-acceptance and self-love. Remember, you are more than just your appearance – your worth lies in your character, accomplishments, and the way you make a difference in the world.

To cultivate a positive body image, prioritize self-care. Engage in activities that promote physical and mental well-being. Regular exercise, such as yoga, walking, or dancing, not only keeps your body strong and flexible but also releases endorphins that boost your mood and overall confidence. Additionally, nourish your body with a balanced diet filled with nutrient-rich foods that support healthy aging. Remember, aging with elegance is not about striving for perfection, but rather about feeling vibrant and energetic.

Surround yourself with a supportive community of women who uplift and inspire you. Seek out friendships with women who value authenticity, inner beauty, and embracing the aging process. Engaging in open and honest conversations about body image and aging can help you gain new perspectives and develop a more positive mindset.

Another important aspect of nurturing a healthy body image is taking care of your skin. Moisturize daily, protect yourself from harmful sun exposure, and explore skincare routines that make you feel pampered and radiant. Remember, aging gracefully is about feeling confident in your skin and allowing your natural beauty to shine through.

Lastly, challenge societal norms and redefine what it means to age with elegance. Embrace your silver strands, wrinkles, and laugh lines as symbols of a life well-lived. Share your wisdom and experiences with younger generations, inspiring them to embrace their years as well.

In conclusion, nurturing a healthy body image is vital for women to age gracefully. By embracing self-acceptance, engaging in self-care, surrounding yourself with a supportive community, and redefining societal norms, you can cultivate a positive mindset and confidently embrace the aging process. Remember, your beauty lies in your uniqueness, and the years ahead are an opportunity to shine even brighter.

Redefining Beauty Standards

In today's society, beauty standards seem to be ever-changing and unattainable for many women. The pressure to look young and flawless can often leave women

feeling self-conscious and inadequate as they age. However, it is time for us to challenge these unrealistic ideals and embrace a new definition of beauty that celebrates the wisdom, strength, and elegance that come with age.

In this subchapter, "Redefining Beauty Standards," we aim to empower women and help them understand that beauty is not confined to youth. Instead, it is a multifaceted concept that evolves with time and experience. We will delve into the societal pressures women face and provide insights on how to break free from the chains of conventional beauty norms.

We will explore the importance of self-acceptance and self-love. Aging is a natural process that we all go through, and it is essential to embrace the changes that come with it. By shifting our mindset and focusing on the positive aspects of aging, we can start to appreciate the unique beauty that each stage of life brings.

Furthermore, we will discuss the significance of inner beauty and how it radiates outwardly. True beauty lies in the confidence, compassion, and kindness that we carry in our hearts. By nurturing our inner selves, we can enhance our outer beauty and inspire others to do the same.

Additionally, we will explore the role of media and its impact on beauty standards. The media often portrays

an unrealistic image of youthfulness and flawlessness, which can be detrimental to women's self-esteem. We will provide practical tips on how to filter and challenge these messages, encouraging women to focus on their individuality and uniqueness.

Throughout this subchapter, we will share inspiring stories of women who have embraced their years with grace and confidence. These stories will serve as a reminder that beauty knows no age limit and that every woman has the power to age gracefully.

In conclusion, "Redefining Beauty Standards" is a subchapter dedicated to helping women break free from the constraints of societal beauty norms. By promoting self-acceptance, inner beauty, and challenging media influences, we aim to inspire women to embrace their years with elegance and confidence. It is time to redefine beauty and celebrate the wisdom and strength that come with age.

Fostering Body Acceptance and Appreciation

In today's society, where unrealistic beauty standards and age-defying expectations prevail, women need to foster body acceptance and appreciation as they age gracefully. The journey of aging should be embraced with confidence and self-love, allowing women to celebrate

every stage of their lives. In this subchapter, we will explore the importance of accepting and appreciating our bodies, providing practical tips and inspiration to help women navigate this transformative process.

First and foremost, it is crucial to recognize that beauty comes in all shapes, sizes, and ages. Instead of comparing ourselves to airbrushed images in magazines or social media, we should focus on cultivating a positive body image that celebrates our uniqueness. Embracing our changing bodies and accepting the natural processes of aging is a powerful step towards self-acceptance.

One effective way to foster body acceptance is through self-care. By prioritizing our physical and mental well-being, we can build a strong foundation for self-love. Engaging in regular exercise, nourishing our bodies with wholesome foods, and practicing mindfulness can all contribute to a healthier body image. When we treat ourselves with kindness and respect, we begin to appreciate the incredible vessel that carries us through life's journey.

Another aspect of fostering body acceptance is challenging societal norms and embracing our individuality. Every woman has her own story, experiences, and wisdom gained through the years. By celebrating our unique qualities and embracing our age, we can inspire others and create a positive ripple effect in our communities. It

is through our authenticity and self-acceptance that we can truly age with elegance.

Additionally, surrounding ourselves with a supportive community of like-minded women can be immensely beneficial. Sharing experiences, struggles, and triumphs creates a sense of belonging and empowers us to embrace our bodies. Engaging in conversations about body positivity and challenging ageist attitudes not only helps us but also encourages others to do the same.

In conclusion, fostering body acceptance and appreciation is vital for women as they age gracefully. It is a journey that requires self-reflection, self-care, and a strong support system. By shifting our focus from external beauty standards to self-love and acceptance, we can embrace our years with elegance and inspire others to do the same. Let us celebrate our bodies, our stories, and the wisdom we have gained, for it is in this acceptance that true beauty and grace reside.

Promoting Healthy Habits for a Radiant Glow

In today's society, there is immense pressure on women to maintain a youthful appearance as they age. However, true elegance lies in embracing the years and taking care of oneself from within. Promoting healthy habits is the key to unlocking a radiant glow that transcends age and

exudes confidence. In this subchapter, we will explore various aspects of self-care and lifestyle choices that can help women age gracefully.

One of the fundamental pillars of promoting a radiant glow is nourishing the body with a healthy diet. Including a variety of fruits, vegetables, whole grains, and lean proteins in your meals can provide the necessary nutrients to support your skin's health. Antioxidant-rich foods, such as blueberries and spinach, can combat free radicals and help slow down the aging process. Additionally, staying hydrated by drinking plenty of water is essential for maintaining supple and glowing skin.

Regular exercise is another vital component of aging gracefully. Engaging in activities that get your heart rate up and boost circulation can improve the appearance of your skin by increasing oxygen and nutrient delivery. Exercise also promotes the release of endorphins, which can enhance your mood and overall well-being.

Taking care of your skin is crucial for maintaining a radiant glow. Establishing a skincare routine that includes cleansing, moisturizing, and protecting your skin from harmful UV rays can help prevent premature aging. Regularly exfoliating your skin can also promote a healthy complexion by removing dead skin cells and revealing fresh, youthful skin.

In addition to physical self-care, promoting a radiant glow also involves nurturing your mental and emotional well-being. Stress can greatly impact your appearance, leading to dull skin and premature aging. Engaging in activities that promote relaxation, such as practicing mindfulness or indulging in a hobby, can help reduce stress levels and improve your overall glow.

Lastly, don't forget the importance of getting enough sleep. A good night's rest allows your body to repair and regenerate, leading to a refreshed and radiant appearance. Establish a consistent sleep schedule and create a relaxing bedtime routine to ensure you are getting the rejuvenating sleep you need.

By adopting these healthy habits, you can promote a radiant glow that transcends the years. Remember, true elegance comes from embracing the journey of aging and taking care of yourself from the inside out. Embrace your years with grace and confidence, and let your inner glow shine through.

CHAPTER 5: EXPLORING NEW PASSIONS AND POSSIBILITIES

Subchapter: Discovering Hobbies and Interests

Introduction:
In the journey of aging gracefully, women must embrace their years with a zest for life. One way to achieve this is by discovering hobbies and interests that bring joy, fulfillment, and a renewed sense of purpose. Engaging in activities that nourish the mind, body, and soul not only enhances overall well-being but also helps in maintaining a positive outlook on life. In this subchapter, we will explore the importance of discovering new hobbies and interests as women age, and how they can contribute to an elegant and fulfilling life.

Embracing Change:
As women age, their lives naturally undergo various transitions. Retirement, empty nests, or changes in health can create voids that were once filled with responsibilities. Discovering new hobbies and interests can help fill these voids, providing avenues

for personal growth, creativity, and self-expression.

Exploring Passions:
Many women have lifelong dreams or interests that may have been put on hold due to career or family commitments. Now is the perfect time to rekindle those passions. Whether it's painting, photography, writing, gardening, or learning a new language, exploring these long-held desires can bring immense joy and fulfillment in the golden years.

Staying Active:
Maintaining an active lifestyle is essential for women as they age. Engaging in physical activities not only promotes physical health but also boosts mental well-being. Whether it's taking up yoga, dancing, swimming, or simply going for regular walks, staying active helps women age gracefully and maintains their youthful vitality.

Connecting with Others:

Discovering new hobbies and interests also provides an opportunity to connect with like-minded individuals. Joining clubs, groups, or classes centered around shared

interests can lead to new friendships, social interactions, and a sense of belonging. These connections play a vital role in combating feelings of loneliness and isolation that can sometimes accompany aging.

Nurturing the Mind and Spirit:
In addition to physical activities, it's equally crucial to engage in hobbies and interests that nurture the mind and spirit. Reading, writing in a journal, meditating, or exploring spirituality can bring a sense of peace, mindfulness, and inner growth. These

practices can help women navigate the emotional and spiritual aspects of aging with grace and elegance.

Conclusion:
Discovering hobbies and interests is an integral part of aging gracefully. It allows women to embrace their years with enthusiasm and a renewed sense of purpose. By exploring passions, staying active, connecting with others, and nurturing the mind and spirit, women can create an elegant and fulfilling life, no matter their age. So, let us embark on this journey of self-discovery together, and embrace the beauty that comes with embracing our years.

Unleashing Creativity Through Artistic Pursuits

In the journey of aging gracefully, one powerful tool that women can utilize is the pursuit of artistic endeavors. Engaging in creative activities not only allows women to express themselves but also unlocks a world of endless possibilities, fostering personal growth and fulfillment. This subchapter explores the transformative power of art in helping women age with elegance and inspire them to embrace their years.

Artistic pursuits offer a unique avenue for self-expression, allowing women to tap into their innermost thoughts and emotions. Whether it's through painting, writing, sculpting, or any other form of artistic expression, women can delve deep into their creativity and find solace, joy, and healing. Art becomes a powerful medium to communicate their experiences, dreams, and aspirations, enabling them to connect with others and leave a lasting legacy.

Engaging in art also allows women to break free from societal expectations and embrace their unique perspectives. As they age, women often face challenges such as loss, changing roles, or a sense of invisibility. However, through artistic pursuits, they can redefine their identities and find renewed purpose. Art offers a platform for self-discovery, empowering women to explore their passions, talents, and abilities that may have been dormant for years.

Moreover, art has therapeutic benefits that can positively impact women's mental and emotional well-being. The act of creating art stimulates the brain, promoting cognitive function and enhancing memory. It serves as a powerful stress reliever, helping women navigate the complexities of aging and find solace in their creative endeavors. Artistic pursuits also provide a sense of accomplishment and self-confidence, boosting self-esteem and fostering a positive outlook on life.

Additionally, art can act as a catalyst for social connection and community building. Joining art classes, workshops, or groups specifically designed for women can create a supportive network where individuals can share their experiences, learn from one another, and form meaningful friendships. Collaborative projects and exhibitions provide opportunities for women to showcase their talents, inspire others, and contribute to the art world.

In conclusion, embracing artistic pursuits opens up a world of possibilities for women to age with elegance and grace. Through art, women can discover their true selves, heal from past experiences, and find new purpose and joy. Whether it's painting, writing, or any other form of creative expression, engaging in art allows women to unleash their creativity, connect with others, and leave a lasting legacy. So, let us encourage and inspire women to

embark on this transformative journey of self-discovery through artistic pursuits.

Exploring New Sports and Fitness Activities

As we age, it is essential to prioritize our physical and mental health. Engaging in regular exercise not only helps us maintain a fit body but also enhances our overall well-being. However, sticking to the same workout routine can become monotonous and less effective over time. That's why it is crucial to explore new sports and fitness activities to keep ourselves motivated and continually challenge our bodies.

Trying out new activities not only adds excitement to our fitness journey but also allows us to discover hidden talents and passions. Whether you are a seasoned athlete or someone who has never been particularly sporty, there is a wide range of activities to choose from, catering to every interest and fitness level.

One of the most popular activities among women of all ages is yoga. Yoga exercises not only improves flexibility and strength but also promotes relaxation and mental clarity. The gentle stretches and breathwork involved in yoga can be particularly beneficial for women looking to age gracefully and maintain a calm, centered mind.

If you prefer a more high-energy workout, why not consider dance classes? From salsa to Zumba, dancing is a fantastic way to improve cardiovascular fitness while having fun and expressing yourself through movement. Dance classes provide an opportunity to socialize, meet new people, and feel the joy of dancing to your favorite tunes.

For those who enjoy being surrounded by nature, hiking, and outdoor activities are excellent options. Exploring new hiking trails or taking up activities like paddleboarding or kayaking can provide a refreshing change of scenery while improving cardiovascular endurance and muscle strength.

Additionally, martial arts such as tai chi or karate are gaining popularity among women due to their numerous health benefits. These activities not only enhance physical fitness but also cultivate discipline, focus, and self-defense skills. They can be especially empowering for women, boosting confidence and promoting a sense of personal security.

No matter which activity you choose, it is important to listen to your body and start slowly, gradually increasing the intensity and duration of your workouts. Remember, the goal is not perfection but progress, and finding joy in the process.

Exploring new sports and fitness activities is an opportunity to step out of our comfort zones, challenge ourselves, and embrace our years with elegance. So, let's lace up our sneakers, try something new, and embark on a journey of self-discovery and fulfillment through the world of sports and fitness.

Engaging in Lifelong Learning

In the journey of life, one constant factor is change. As women, we navigate our way through various stages, facing different challenges and embracing new opportunities. As we age, it becomes even more crucial to prioritize our personal growth and development. Engaging in lifelong learning is an essential aspect of aging gracefully and embracing our years with elegance.

Lifelong learning is not confined to the walls of a classroom or limited to a certain age group. It is a mindset, a commitment to continuously seek knowledge, explore new ideas, and develop new skills. By investing in our intellectual and emotional growth, we empower ourselves to face the challenges that come with aging and embrace the beauty that each stage of life brings.

One of the most significant benefits of engaging in lifelong learning is the expansion of our horizons. It allows us to explore different interests, discover hidden tal

ents, and develop new passions. Whether it's learning a new language, exploring the arts, or delving into history, each new pursuit broadens our perspective and enriches our lives.

Moreover, lifelong learning enhances our mental well-being. Studies have shown that actively engaging in intellectual activities can delay cognitive decline and reduce the risk of developing age-related diseases such as dementia. By challenging our minds and keeping them active, we maintain our mental sharpness, memory, and overall cognitive abilities.

Another aspect of lifelong learning is the opportunity for personal growth and self-discovery. As women, we are constantly evolving, and by engaging in learning, we nurture our personal development. It allows us to reflect on our values, beliefs, and desires, enabling us to make informed decisions and live a more fulfilling life.

Furthermore, engaging in lifelong learning strengthens our sense of empowerment and independence. It equips us with the knowledge and skills necessary to navigate the ever-changing world around us. Whether it's adapting to new technologies, understanding financial matters, or staying informed about current events, being well-informed empowers us to make confident choices and actively participate in society.

As women who aspire to age gracefully, we must embrace the concept of lifelong learning. Let us break free from the notion that learning is limited to a specific period of our lives or confined to formal education. Instead, let us adopt a mindset of curiosity, exploration, and growth. By engaging in lifelong learning, we empower ourselves to live vibrant, fulfilling lives, embracing the wisdom and beauty that comes with each passing year.

Pursuing Dreams and Ambitions

In the journey of aging gracefully, women must recognize and nourish their dreams and ambitions. As we age, it is easy to fall into the trap of thinking that our dreams are no longer attainable or that we have missed our opportunities. However, it is never too late to pursue our passions and embrace the endless possibilities that life has to offer.

Dreams and ambitions are the fuel that ignites our spirits and keeps us motivated. They give us a sense of purpose and fulfillment, helping us navigate the challenges that come with aging. It is essential to remember that dreams do not have an expiry date; on the contrary, they become even more meaningful as we grow older.

One of the keys to pursuing dreams and ambitions is to acknowledge and embrace the wisdom and experience

that comes with age. Throughout our lives, we have accumulated a wealth of knowledge and skills that can be applied to any pursuit. Whether it is starting a new business, learning a new language, or exploring a new hobby, our life experiences give us a unique advantage and a solid foundation to build upon.

Another crucial aspect of pursuing dreams and ambitions is cultivating a supportive network of like-minded women. Connecting with others who share similar aspirations can provide inspiration, encouragement, and an invaluable source of guidance. Surrounding ourselves with empowering and uplifting women can help us overcome self-doubt and increase our confidence in pursuing our dreams.

It is also important to let go of societal expectations and embrace the freedom that comes with aging. As women, we may have spent a significant portion of our lives fulfilling the expectations of others, be it as mothers, daughters, or caregivers. Now is the time to prioritize our desires and passions. Aging offers us the opportunity to rediscover ourselves, explore new interests, and redefine success on our terms.

In conclusion, pursuing dreams and ambitions is an essential aspect of aging with elegance. By nourishing our dreams, embracing our experiences, and building a supportive network, we can continue to grow and thrive

throughout our lives. Let us remind ourselves that our dreams are timeless and that we deserve to pursue them with passion and vigor. Embrace the beauty of your years and allow your dreams to guide you toward a life filled with purpose and fulfillment.

Reinventing Career Pathways

In today's world, women are breaking barriers, shattering glass ceilings, and making their mark in every industry. Gone are the days when retirement meant the end of a woman's professional journey. Instead, aging gracefully now involves reinventing career pathways and embracing new opportunities that align with personal passions and skills.

Reinventing career pathways can be an exciting and fulfilling endeavor for women as they navigate the later stages of their lives. It offers a chance to explore untapped potential, discover hidden talents, and embark on a new journey that brings joy and meaning. Whether it's starting a business, pursuing a creative endeavor, or finding purpose in volunteer work, there are endless possibilities for women to continue growing and contributing to society.

One of the key aspects of reinventing career pathways is identifying one's unique strengths and interests. It's an

opportunity to reflect on past experiences, skills gained, and the knowledge accumulated over the years. This self-reflection process allows women to determine their true passions and find alignment between their professional aspirations and personal values.

Moreover, reinventing career pathways can also involve acquiring new skills or further developing existing ones. With the advancement of technology and the availability of online courses, it has never been easier for women to expand their knowledge and embrace new fields. From digital marketing to graphic design, from coding to entrepreneurship, the possibilities are endless. Embracing lifelong learning not only keeps the mind sharp but also opens doors to exciting new opportunities.

Furthermore, reinventing career pathways often requires a shift in mindset. Women need to overcome any self-limiting beliefs or societal expectations that may hinder their progress. Aging gracefully means embracing the wisdom and experience accumulated over the years and using it as a powerful tool to navigate new professional ventures. Confidence, resilience, and adaptability become essential traits in this journey of reinvention.

Lastly, reinventing career pathways is not solely about personal growth and fulfillment; it is also about making a positive impact on the world. Many women choose to focus their reinvented careers on giving back to their

communities, mentoring younger generations, or championing causes close to their hearts. By combining their skills and passions with a sense of purpose, these women inspire others and create a legacy that goes beyond professional success.

In conclusion, reinventing career pathways is a transformative opportunity for women to age gracefully. It allows them to tap into their unique strengths, explore new possibilities, and continue making a difference in their own lives and the world around them. By embracing this journey of reinvention, women can inspire others and prove that age is not a barrier to success, but rather a stepping stone towards a more fulfilling and purposeful life.

Starting a New Business or Venture

As women, embracing our years means continually exploring new opportunities and embracing change. Starting a new business or venture is an exciting and empowering way to channel our passions and skills, while also inspiring others and leaving a lasting impact on the world.

When it comes to starting a new business or venture, the first step is to identify your passion. What drives you? What are you truly passionate about? This could be any

thing from a hobby to a cause you deeply care about. By aligning your business with your passion, you will find the motivation and determination needed to turn your dreams into reality.

Next, it is crucial to conduct thorough market research. Understand your target audience and their needs. What problems can your business solve? By gaining a clear understanding of your potential customers, you can tailor your products or services to meet their specific demands.

Developing a comprehensive business plan is essential for success. Your plan should outline your goals, strategies, and financial projections. It will serve as a roadmap, guiding you through the initial stages of your venture. Additionally, a well-structured business plan will help you secure funding and attract potential investors.

Networking is another key component when starting a new business. Connect with other like-minded individuals, join professional organizations, and attend industry events. Building a strong network will not only provide you with valuable advice and support, but it can also lead to potential partnerships and collaborations that can accelerate your business's growth.

As women, it is crucial to embrace technology and the digital world. Establishing a strong online presence through a website and social media platforms can significantly expand your reach and attract a wider customer base. Utilize digital marketing strategies to effectively promote your business and engage with your audience.

Lastly, remember that starting a new business or venture is a journey. It may come with challenges and setbacks, but perseverance and resilience are key. Embrace each experience as an opportunity to learn and grow, and never be afraid to seek guidance from mentors or business advisors. With determination and a positive mindset, you can create a successful and fulfilling business venture that not only helps you age gracefully but also empowers and inspires other women to do the same.

In conclusion, starting a new business or venture is a powerful way for women to embrace their years with elegance. By identifying our passions, conducting market research, developing a solid business plan, networking, utilizing technology, and embracing resilience, we can create businesses that not only contribute to our personal growth but also inspire others to embrace their journey of aging gracefully.

Leaving a Legacy Through Philanthropy

In the journey of life, it is essential for women to not only age gracefully but also leave a lasting impact on the world. One powerful way to achieve this is through philanthropy. Giving back to causes and communities that hold meaning in our hearts not only enriches the lives of others but also becomes a legacy that will be remembered long after we are gone.

Philanthropy is not limited to financial contributions alone. It encompasses a wide range of actions, including volunteering time, offering expertise, and advocating for social change. As women, we have the power to make a difference in the lives of those less fortunate, and by doing so, we can inspire others to follow in our footsteps.

Aging gracefully is about embracing the wisdom and experiences that come with growing older. It is about recognizing the value we hold and using it to create positive change in the world around us. Philanthropy offers a unique opportunity to leave a legacy that aligns with our values and passions.

When considering philanthropic endeavors, it is important to reflect on the causes that resonate with us personally. Whether it is supporting education, healthcare, environmental conservation, or advocating for women's

rights, it is crucial to find a cause that ignites our passion and motivates us to take action.

By engaging in philanthropy, we not only help others but also experience personal fulfillment and a sense of purpose. The act of giving back can bring joy, satisfaction, and a renewed sense of gratitude for the blessings we have in our own lives. It allows us to connect with like-minded individuals, forms meaningful relationships, and build a network of support that can further our impact.

Leaving a legacy through philanthropy is not confined to the wealthy or influential. Every woman can make a difference, regardless of her financial situation. It is the intention behind our actions, the love, and compassion we bring to the table, that truly leaves a lasting impact.

In this subchapter, we will explore various ways in which women can engage in philanthropy, whether it is through donations, volunteering, or using their skills and knowledge to make a difference. We will also delve into the profound effects that philanthropy has on our well-being and the lives of those we touch.

Together, let us embrace the power of philanthropy and leave a legacy that inspires generations to come. Let us

age with elegance and grace, knowing that our impact on the world will continue long after we are gone.

CHAPTER 6: EMBRACING AGING WITH GRACE AND WISDOM

Embodying Graceful Aging

As women, we have the power to age with grace and elegance. It is not just about looking youthful, but about embracing the wisdom and experiences that come with each passing year. In this subchapter, we will explore the various ways in which we can embody graceful aging and inspire others to do the same.

1. Cultivating a Positive Mindset: Aging gracefully begins with our mindset. Instead of focusing on the physical changes that come with age, we can shift our attention toward the wisdom, strength, and resilience we have gained over the years. By embracing a positive mindset,

we can radiate confidence and inspire others to do the same.

2. Prioritizing Self-Care: Taking care of ourselves becomes even more important as we age. Engaging in regular exercise, maintaining a healthy diet, and getting enough rest are all crucial

for our overall well-being. By prioritizing self-care, we can feel and look our best, enhancing our graceful aging journey.

3. Nurturing Relationships: Building strong and meaningful relationships is vital in every stage of life. As we age, it becomes even more important to surround ourselves with loved ones who support and inspire us. By cultivating deep connections, we can create a sense of fulfillment and joy, making the aging process more enjoyable.

4. Embracing New Challenges: Aging gracefully does not mean avoiding challenges; it means embracing them with open arms. As we age, we should seek opportunities for personal growth and learning. Whether it's trying a new hobby, pursuing further education, or exploring new interests, stepping out of our comfort zones keeps our minds sharp and our spirits vibrant.

5. Celebrating Inner Beauty: True beauty radiates from within, and as we age, it becomes even more appar

ent. Embrace your unique qualities, celebrate your accomplishments, and showcase your inner beauty to the world. By doing so, you inspire other women to appreciate their uniqueness and age gracefully.

In conclusion, embodying graceful aging is a journey of self-discovery and self-care. By cultivating a positive mindset, prioritizing self-care, nurturing relationships, embracing new challenges, and celebrating inner beauty, we can inspire other women to age gracefully. Let us embrace our years with elegance, wisdom, and a zest for life, showing the world that age is just a number.

Cultivating Inner Peace and Serenity

In the hustle and bustle of our daily lives, it's easy to forget the importance of nurturing our inner selves. As women, we often find ourselves juggling multiple roles and responsibilities, leaving little time for self-care and reflection. However, as we age gracefully, it becomes increasingly vital to cultivate inner peace and serenity to navigate life's challenges with grace and elegance.

Inner peace and serenity are not elusive concepts reserved for the spiritually enlightened; they are attainable states of mind that we can cultivate within ourselves. By prioritizing our mental and emotional well-being, we

can navigate the aging process with grace, embracing the wisdom and beauty that come with each passing year.

One of the most effective ways to cultivate inner peace is through the practice of mindfulness. Mindfulness involves being fully present in the moment, paying attention to our thoughts, feelings, and sensations without judgment. By cultivating mindfulness, we can let go of worries about the future or regrets about the past, allowing ourselves to experience genuine tranquility and contentment.

Another powerful tool to cultivate inner peace is the practice of self-compassion. As women, we often hold ourselves to impossibly high standards and berate ourselves for perceived failures. However, by treating ourselves with kindness, understanding, and forgiveness, we can create a nurturing environment within our hearts. Self-compassion enables us to accept ourselves fully, flaws and all, and fosters a sense of inner peace and serenity.

In addition to mindfulness and self-compassion, finding activities that bring us joy and relaxation can also help cultivate inner peace. Whether it's taking a leisurely walk in nature, practicing yoga, painting, or listening to calming music, carving out time for activities that nourish our souls is crucial. These moments of solace allow us

to recharge, rejuvenate, and reconnect with our inner selves.

Lastly, creating a supportive community of like-minded women can significantly contribute to our inner peace and serenity. Surrounding ourselves with individuals who uplift and inspire us can provide a sense of belonging and support as we navigate the ups and downs of life. Sharing our experiences, joys, and challenges with others can bring a profound sense of connection and inner peace.

As women, aging gracefully is not just about the external appearance; it's about nurturing our inner selves and cultivating a sense of inner peace and serenity. By incorporating mindfulness, self-compassion, joyful activities, and supportive communities into our lives, we can embrace the years with elegance and grace, becoming shining examples for others to follow. Remember, cultivating inner peace is a lifelong journey, and each step we take brings us closer to a life filled with tranquility and contentment.

Practicing Patience and Compassion

In the journey of aging gracefully, one of the most valuable qualities a woman can cultivate is the art of practicing patience and compassion. As the years go by, we

often find ourselves facing new challenges and changes - both in our physical appearance and in our daily lives. It is during these times that patience and compassion become essential tools to help us navigate through this chapter of our lives with grace and dignity.

Firstly, let us explore the importance of patience. As we age, our bodies naturally go through various transformations, and it can be tempting to become frustrated or disheartened by these changes. However, by practicing patience, we can learn to accept and embrace these transformations, understanding that they are a natural part of the aging process. Patience allows us to approach these changes with a sense of serenity and self-acceptance, enabling us to appreciate the beauty that comes with each passing year.

Furthermore, compassion plays a crucial role in helping women age gracefully. As we grow older, it is not uncommon to encounter health issues or limitations that may require assistance from others. By cultivating compassion, we learn to be kind and understanding toward ourselves and those around us. We become more willing to ask for help when needed and more attuned to the needs of others, fostering a sense of community and support as we navigate the challenges of aging.

Practicing patience and compassion also extends beyond our physical well-being. It involves cultivating patience

with ourselves as we adapt to new stages of life, such as retirement or becoming empty nesters. It means showing compassion towards ourselves as we reflect on past accomplishments and set new goals for the future. By doing so, we create an atmosphere of self-acceptance and self-love that radiates outwards, inspiring those around us and empowering them to embrace their years with elegance.

In conclusion, the subchapter "Practicing Patience and Compassion" highlights the significance of these virtues in helping women age gracefully. By nurturing patience, we learn to accept and appreciate the changes that come with aging. By cultivating compassion, we foster a sense of understanding and unity, both within ourselves and within our communities. Through these practices, we can transform the journey of aging into one of growth, fulfillment, and elegance.

Embracing Wisdom and Life Experience

In the journey of life, aging is an inevitable part that each one of us must face. Rather than viewing it with trepidation, we should strive to embrace the wisdom and life experience that comes with growing older. This subchapter aims to inspire women to age gracefully and appreciate the richness that each passing year brings.

As women, we often find ourselves bombarded with societal pressures to maintain a youthful appearance. However, the true essence of aging lies not in the lines on our faces or the graying of our hair, but in the depth of knowledge and experiences, we have accumulated over the years. It is important to shift our focus from external appearances to the inner growth that accompanies the passage of time.

Wisdom is not something that can be acquired overnight; it is a result of a lifetime of experiences, victories, and challenges. By embracing our life experiences, we can tap into a wellspring of knowledge that allows us to navigate the complexities of the world with grace and resilience. Our years spent juggling careers, raising families, and overcoming obstacles have equipped us with a unique perspective that should be celebrated.

Aging gracefully also entails accepting and cherishing the changes that occur within our bodies. Our physical appearance may change, but it is a testament to the strength and endurance we have exhibited throughout our lives. Rather than viewing wrinkles and grey hair as signs of decline, we should embrace them as badges of honor that signify the resilience and beauty of a life well-lived.

Furthermore, as we grow older, it becomes increasingly important to prioritize self-care and invest in our overall

well-being. This includes nourishing our minds, bodies, and spirits through activities that bring joy, such as pursuing hobbies, engaging in regular exercise, and cultivating meaningful relationships. By taking care of ourselves, we can continue to thrive and contribute to the world around us.

In conclusion, the subchapter "Embracing Wisdom and Life Experience" seeks to inspire women to appreciate the journey of aging and the wealth of knowledge and experiences it brings. By shifting our focus from external appearances to inner growth, accepting the changes in our bodies, and prioritizing self-care, we can truly embrace our years with elegance and grace. Let us celebrate the wisdom and life experience that make us unique and empower ourselves to live our best lives, regardless of age.

Subchapter: Inspiring Other Women to Embrace Their Years

Introduction:
As women, we often find ourselves grappling with societal pressures and expectations surrounding aging. However, the key to aging gracefully lies not in trying to defy the passing years, but in embracing them with elegance and confidence. In this subchapter, we will explore

the importance of inspiring other women to embrace their years, and how doing so can transform our own lives and those around us.

1. Celebrating Wisdom and Experience:
One of the most significant aspects of aging gracefully is recognizing the wealth of wisdom and experience that comes with each passing year. By sharing our knowledge and insights, we can inspire other women to value their unique journeys and view the aging process as an opportunity for growth and self-discovery.

2. Redefining Beauty:
In a culture that often equates youth with beauty, it is essential to challenge these narrow definitions and redefine what it means to be beautiful. By embracing our years, we can inspire other women to embrace their unique beauty, emphasizing the importance of self-care, self-love, and nurturing our inner selves.

3. Embracing Change:
Aging is a natural part of life, and with it comes inevitable changes in our bodies and lifestyles. By embracing these changes

and adapting gracefully, we can inspire other women to do the same. By encouraging a positive attitude towards change, we can help women navigate the challenges that come with aging, empowering them to embrace new opportunities and find joy in every stage of life.

4. Cultivating Confidence and Empowerment:
Inspiring other women to embrace their years involves cultivating confidence and empowering them to live their lives to the fullest. By sharing our stories of personal growth and resilience, we can encourage women to step into their power and pursue their dreams, no matter their age. Emphasizing the importance of self-belief and self-acceptance, we can inspire women to overcome societal limitations and live authentically.

Conclusion:
In this subchapter, we have explored the significance of inspiring other women to embrace their years. By celebrating wisdom, redefining beauty, embracing change, and cultivating confidence, we can help women age with grace and elegance. As we inspire others, we also uplift ourselves, creating a supportive community of women who celebrate the beauty and strength that comes with each passing year. Let us embark on this journey together, inspiring one another to embrace our years and live our lives to the fullest.

Becoming a Role Model for Other Women

In today's society, where the emphasis on youth and beauty prevails, women must embrace their years and age gracefully. As women, we have a unique opportunity to become role models for others, inspiring them to navigate the aging process with elegance and confidence.

By embracing our journey and sharing our wisdom, we can empower and uplift other women, fostering a community of support and celebration.

First and foremost, it is important to recognize that beauty transcends age. Our physical appearance may change over time, but true beauty radiates from within. By nourishing our minds, bodies, and spirits, we can exude a captivating aura that defies societal expectations. As role models, we can encourage other women to prioritize self-care and self-love, reminding them that their value is not determined by their outward appearance.

Furthermore, aging gracefully involves embracing the wisdom and experiences that come with each passing year. As we accumulate knowledge and life lessons, we become reservoirs of wisdom that can guide and inspire others. By sharing our stories and insights, we can help women navigate the challenges and triumphs of aging, offering them guidance and support along the way.

Additionally, it is essential to redefine societal norms and expectations surrounding aging. As role models, we can challenge ageist beliefs and inspire women to rewrite their narratives. By celebrating our accomplishments, pursuing our passions, and embracing new challenges, we can demonstrate that age is just a number. Through our actions, we can show other women that life con

tinues to offer opportunities for growth and fulfillment, regardless of age.

Lastly, becoming a role model for other women means fostering a sense of community and sisterhood. By building connections and supporting one another, we create a network of empowerment and encouragement. Together, we can overcome societal pressures and redefine what it means to age with elegance. By sharing our journeys, offering advice, and celebrating each other's successes, we can inspire a generation of women to embrace their years and live their lives to the fullest.

In conclusion, as women, we have the power to become role models for others and help them navigate the aging process with elegance. By embracing our journey, sharing our wisdom, redefining societal norms, and fostering a sense of community, we can inspire women to age gracefully. Let us stand together, celebrate our years, and empower each other to embrace the beauty and wisdom that come over time.

Sharing Stories of Empowerment and Resilience

In the subchapter "Sharing Stories of Empowerment and Resilience" from the book "Aging with Elegance: Inspiring Women to Embrace Their Years," we delve into the

remarkable journeys of women who have learned to age gracefully, finding strength, empowerment, and resilience along the way. These stories are meant to inspire and uplift women who are seeking guidance on how to navigate the aging process with grace and confidence.

This subchapter serves as a reminder that age is just a number and that every woman has the potential to embrace her years with elegance. By sharing these stories, we create a safe space for women to connect, learn from one another, and find solace in the experiences of others who have faced similar challenges.

Through these narratives of empowerment and resilience, we explore the diverse paths women have taken to cultivate a sense of self-worth, inner strength, and confidence as they age. From overcoming societal expectations and stereotypes to flourishing in their personal and professional lives, these women have defied the limitations often associated with aging.

We hear from women who have reinvented themselves in their later years, discovering new passions, hobbies, and careers that bring them joy and fulfillment. Their stories highlight the importance of embracing change, stepping out of one's comfort zone, and embracing one's true potential.

Additionally, we explore how these women have nurtured their physical, mental, and emotional well-being. From adopting healthy lifestyle habits to cultivating meaningful relationships and finding purpose in their daily lives, they demonstrate that aging gracefully begins from within.

This subchapter offers practical advice and actionable tips for women to enhance their self-care routines, boost their confidence, and develop a resilient mindset. It encourages readers to celebrate their accomplishments, focus on their strengths, and embrace the wisdom that comes with age.

As women, we are all on this journey together, and by sharing our stories of empowerment and resilience, we can inspire and support one another as we navigate the challenges and joys of aging. By embracing our years with elegance, we can live our lives to the fullest, shining as examples for future generations of women.

Supporting and Uplifting Women of All Ages

In today's society, women are often bombarded with messages about the importance of youth and beauty. However, the true essence of a woman lies in her wisdom, strength, and resilience, regardless of her age. Aging with elegance is about embracing every stage of

life and recognizing the unique beauty that comes with it. This subchapter aims to inspire and support women of all ages in their journey of graceful aging.

One of the key aspects of embracing the aging process is self-care. As women, we often prioritize the needs of others above our own, but it is vital to remember that self-care is not selfish. Making time for ourselves, whether it's through exercise, hobbies, meditation, or simply pampering ourselves, can have a profound impact on our overall well-being. By taking care of ourselves, we are better equipped to support and uplift those around us.

Another important element in aging with elegance is cultivating a positive mindset. Society often perpetuates negative stereotypes about aging, but it's crucial to challenge these beliefs and instead focus on the opportunities and wisdom that come with age. By embracing our years, we can inspire younger generations and serve as role models for women who are navigating their path.

Supporting and uplifting women of all ages also means fostering a sense of community. By connecting with other women, we can share our experiences, offer advice, and provide a shoulder to lean on during challenging times. This support network can be instrumental in helping us navigate the various stages of life, whether it's through motherhood, career transitions, or the chal

lenges that come with aging. Together, we can empower each other to embrace our years with grace and dignity.

Lastly, it is essential to celebrate our accomplishments and embrace our individuality. Each woman has a unique story to tell, and our age should never define us or limit our potential. By acknowledging and celebrating our achievements, we can inspire others and show them that age is just a number.

In conclusion, supporting and uplifting women of all ages is essential in helping them age gracefully. By prioritizing self-care, cultivating a positive mindset, fostering a sense of community, and celebrating our accomplishments, we can inspire and empower women to embrace their years with elegance and confidence. Let us encourage each other on this journey and redefine societal expectations of aging. Together, we can create a world where women of all ages are celebrated for the incredible individuals they are.

Conclusion: Embracing the Journey of Aging with Elegance

As women, our journey through life is a beautiful tapestry woven with experiences, triumphs, and challenges. One of the most profound and inevitable aspects of this journey is the process of aging. While society often paints a negative picture of growing older, it is time for us to change the narrative. Aging is a gift, an opportunity to embrace our years with grace, confidence, and elegance.

In this book, "Aging with Elegance: Inspiring Women to Embrace Their Years," we have explored various aspects of aging, from physical changes to emotional well-being, from self-care to finding purpose. Throughout these pages, we have discovered that aging gracefully is not about defying the passage of time; it is about embracing it wholeheartedly and making the most of every stage in our lives.

The journey of aging with elegance begins with self-acceptance and self-love. We must acknowledge and appreciate the unique beauty that comes with every passing year. Our wrinkles, gray hair, and changing bodies tell a story of resilience, wisdom, and experience. Rather than trying to hide or deny these signs of aging, we should celebrate them as badges of honor.

Furthermore, taking care of ourselves becomes paramount as we age. This includes nourishing our bodies with healthy foods, engaging in regular exercise, and prioritizing mental and emotional well-being. Self-care rituals, such as meditation, journaling, or simply indulging in a bubble bath, can help us cultivate a deeper connection with ourselves and nurture our souls.

But aging gracefully is not just about our physical and emotional well-being; it is also about finding purpose and embracing new opportunities. As we age, we have the wisdom and experience to make meaningful contributions to our communities, families, and the world. Whether it is volunteering, pursuing a new hobby, starting a business, or mentoring younger women, we have the power to make a difference.

In conclusion, Thank you for reading this book. Let us embrace the journey of aging with elegance. Let us defy societal expectations and show the world that growing older is not something to be feared but something to be celebrated. By loving ourselves, taking care of our bodies and minds, and finding purpose, we can inspire other women to do the same. Together, we can create a society where aging is seen as a beautiful and empowering process. Embrace your years, for they are your greatest asset.

Printed in Dunstable, United Kingdom

64202891R00057